MENTAL HEALTH BOOST THROUGH EXCISE

A Holistic Approach to Abundant Mental Wellness, Unleashing the Power of Exercise, Positive Living, and Personal Transformation"

Carl E. Ross

Table of content

INTRODUCTION

Emma was a young lady who struggled to overcome the shadows of fear that surrounded her daily. She resided in the charming village of Serenity Springs. She was having a hard time finding some peace of mind until she came across a book that was titled "Mindful Movements: A Mental Health Boost through Exercise." Intrigued, Emma dove into its pages, where she found that she was about to go on an adventure that would completely change her life.

A tale of hope via physical exercise was revealed in the book, which was written by the well-known psychologist Dr. Katherine Wells. The idea that physical activity is beneficial not just to one's physical health but also to one's mental health was one that Emma enthusiastically embraced. She set off on a trip that would completely transform her life, and she was motivated to do so by the book's advice.

In the beginning, Emma's feet were hesitant, and her heart was filled with uncertainty. On the other hand, she learned that the therapeutic rhythm of her own breath and the healing power of movement were both revealed to her with each new chapter. She started incorporating some kind of physical activity into her daily routine, such as going for morning walks or participating in yoga classes. This helped her break down the barricades that anxiety had built up around her.

As Emma immersed herself in the lessons contained in the book, she discovered that she had not only become physically stronger but also emotionally tougher. The endorphins created during her exercises became her friends in the struggle against stress, and the rhythmic rhythms of exercise became a meditative dance that quieted the turmoil inside.

Her sudden power didn't go unnoticed by people around her. Friends and family noticed a change in Emma - a flowering of confidence and a brilliant light that surpassed the simply physical. Dr. Katherine Wells, pleased by Emma's devotion, came out to convey her thanks, forging a link that spanned the gap between author and reader.

Emma's tale became an inspiration inside Serenity Springs, starting a movement of its own. Local community centers embraced the notion of holistic well-being, holding fitness courses aimed to promote mental health. The ripple effect of Emma's metamorphosis stretched beyond the village, mirroring the book's message in faraway corners where people sought a light of hope.

The last chapter of "Mindful Movements" reinforced the concept that Emma had absorbed — the road toward mental wellness was continual, an ever-evolving discipline. The book finished with an invitation to share one's tale, a monument to the communal power that may be garnered from shared experiences.

As the final page flipped, Emma stood in the golden warmth of the sunset, a symbol of tenacity and self-discovery. Through the knowledge taught by "Mindful Movements," she not only survived the shadows of worry but emerged as a light of encouragement for others on their transforming journeys.

Welcome to MindFit Mastery

where the search for mental well-being meets the art of holistic empowerment. In a society defined by ongoing difficulties, MindFit Mastery emerges as a beacon of total well-being. Our commitment is to lead you on a transforming path towards mental resilience and energy.

The Impact of Holistic Approaches on Mental Health:

In an age when mental health is vital, the relevance of holistic treatments cannot be emphasized. MindFit Mastery addresses the significant effect of integrating physical, emotional, and spiritual well-being into the fabric of mental health techniques. Embracing a holistic mentality goes beyond traditional techniques, giving a deeper knowledge of the interconnection that forms our mental well-being. Discover how a balanced combination of mindfulness, nutrition, and self-discovery may drive you toward lasting mental fortitude.

Setting the Stage for Your Mental Wellness Journey:

Embark on a transforming trip as MindFit Mastery sets the scene for your mental health quest. We realize that genuine well-being exceeds the absence of sickness; it's about flourishing in every element of life. Through highly chosen information, individualized programs, and a supportive community, we give you the tools to unleash your mental potential. Whether you're starting your journey or wanting to develop your practice, MindFit Mastery provides a path personalized to your particular requirements.

Chapter 1: The Synergy of Exercise and Mental Health:

Understanding the Mind-Body Connection

In our fast-paced environment, the necessity of mental health cannot be overstated. Chapter 1 looks into the delicate links between exercise and mental well-being, showing the astonishing synergy that happens within the mind-body connection.

This chapter examines the scientific underpinnings of how physical exercise helps mental health, highlighting the multiple systems that contribute to this symbiotic link. Readers will get a complete understanding of how exercise influences neurotransmitters, hormones, and other physiological factors, ultimately altering one's mental state.

The narrative weaves through the psychological intricacies, exposing the great effect of regular exercise on stress reduction, mood enhancement, and cognitive function. By providing a foundation rooted in scientific principles, this chapter sets the stage for a deeper look at the customized strategies individuals could take to enhance their mental well-being via conscious physical activity.

Scientific Insights on Exercise and Neurotransmitters

Dive into the complexities of neurotransmitters and their dynamic relationship with exercise in Chapter

2. Uncover the brain magic that occurs when you engage in physical activity, changing neurotransmitter release and reception.

This section looks into the role of serotonin, dopamine, and endorphins - the brain's chemical messengers – and how their levels are affected by exercise. Readers will obtain a complete comprehension of how these neurotransmitters contribute to mood regulation, stress management, and overall mental resilience.

The chapter not only examines the favorable results but also delves into the prospective downsides, offering a balanced perspective on the delicate balance of neurotransmitter management. By demystifying the science underpinning exercise and neurotransmitters, readers will be supplied with the knowledge to make informed choices for their mental well-being.

Tailoring Your Exercise Routine for Mental Well-being

Building on the scientific foundation developed in the past chapters, Chapter 3 instructs readers on the skill of constructing a fitness regimen that perfectly caters to mental well-being. This section underlines the benefits of tailored therapies, emphasizing that each individual's mental health journey is unique.

Readers will discover practical strategies to link their fitness plans with their mental health goals. From the intensity and duration of workouts to the choice of activities, this chapter presents real recommendations to help individuals develop an exercise routine that not only suits their physical health but also nurtures their mental resilience.

Incorporating evidence-based recommendations, this chapter gives as a practical guide for readers to traverse the broad range of exercise choices. Whether it's the tranquility of yoga, the invigoration of cardiovascular exercise, or the strength-building benefits of resistance training, this chapter urges readers to take a holistic approach to mental well-being via intentional and tailored physical activity.

These chapters give the groundwork for a transformative journey, teaching readers with both knowledge and practical skills to harness the synergistic potential of exercise and mental health, encouraging a strong and resilient mind-body connection.

Chapter 2: Positive Living for Mental Resilience

In the search for mental resilience, Chapter 2 dives into the enormous effect of optimism on the human brain, dissecting the science underlying its transformational power. Understanding the complicated relationship between positive and mental well-being gives a basis for cultivating a resilient attitude.

The Science of Positivity and its Influence on the Brain

Embarking on a trip into the neuroscience of optimism, we investigate the subtle workings of the brain when exposed to positive stimuli. Scientific study highlights the release of neurotransmitters including dopamine and serotonin, which play key roles in regulating mood and increasing cognitive abilities. Unraveling the delicate dance of neurons, this chapter navigates the neurological terrain, revealing how a positive mentality may change brain circuits and reinforce mental resilience.

Cultivating a Positive Mindset in Daily Life

Shaping a happy mentality demands purposeful efforts in our everyday lives. This section leads readers through practical tactics and practices that help to generate optimism. From mindfulness techniques to gratitude rituals, each method is anchored on psychological principles aimed at boosting optimism and resilience. By incorporating these tactics into everyday routines, people may empower themselves to face life's problems with a constructive and cheerful view.

Integrating Positivity into Relationships and Work

Positivity goes beyond individual well-being; it is a strong force inside interpersonal ties and professional efforts. This part analyzes the rippling effects of a happy mentality on relationships and work situations. From cultivating open communication to maintaining a collaborative culture, embracing optimism promotes cooperation, creativity, and overall pleasure. Moreover, the chapter gives ideas about addressing obstacles, disagreements, and disappointments through a positive perspective, increasing adaptation and resilience in both personal and professional realms.

As we explore the subtleties of positive living, this chapter offers as a blueprint for persons looking to reinforce their mental resilience. Grounded in scientific knowledge, the investigation of positivity's influence on the brain, paired with practical solutions for everyday living and relationships, gives readers with skills to negotiate the complexity of the contemporary world. By embracing the science and art of positive living, people may create mental resilience that allows them to flourish in the face of adversity.

Chapter 3: MindFit Nutrition: Fueling Your Brain for Optimal Performance

In today's fast-paced environment, when cognitive demands are greater than ever, knowing the underlying relationship between diet and mental health is crucial. In this chapter, we dig into MindFit Nutrition, investigating the complex ways dietary elements impact mental well-being and how constructing a Mind-Boosting Diet may increase cognitive function.

Nutritional Factors Affecting Mental Health

The proverb "You are what you eat" takes on additional relevance when contemplating its influence on mental health. Numerous research have underlined the relationship between diet and mood, cognition, and general mental well-being. From the omega-3 fatty acids needed for brain formation to the vast variety of vitamins and minerals supporting neurotransmitter activity, each nutrient performs a key role.

Explore with us the intricate interaction of nutrients like B vitamins, antioxidants, and amino acids, understanding the science underlying their effect on neurotransmitter synthesis and brain function. As we negotiate this nutritional environment, you'll acquire insights into how shortages or imbalances might lead to diseases such as anxiety, depression, and cognitive decline.

Building a Mind-Boosting Diet

Crafting a diet that promotes healthy brain function entails more than tracking calories. Our investigation extends to the notion of a Mind-Boosting Diet – a carefully chosen mix of foods that support cognitive wellness. From consuming brain-friendly superfoods to recognizing the relevance of a balanced macronutrient composition, we present practical recommendations for effectively integrating these nutritional concepts into your everyday life.

Discover the interplay of complex carbs, lean proteins, and healthy fats in preserving mental clarity and attention. Unearth the advantages of adopting a range of colorful fruits and vegetables, rich in antioxidants that counteract oxidative stress and inflammation, both of which have direct consequences for cognitive function.

Hydration and its Impact on Cognitive Function

Amidst talks about diet, the significance of hydration frequently takes a backseat. However, its role in supporting good cognitive function cannot be emphasized. We dig into the science of hydration, studying how appropriate water consumption affects neurotransmitter production, cerebral blood flow, and general brain function.

Join us as we explore the subtle indicators of dehydration and its possible influence on cognitive functions. Gain practical insights into building a hydration program that matches your Mind-Boosting Diet, guaranteeing continuous mental clarity throughout the day.

In this chapter, we not only explore the science behind MindFit Nutrition but also provide you with specific methods to increase your cognitive well-being. Embrace the road toward maximum mental performance by understanding the synergistic link between your food choices and the extraordinary powers of your mind.

Chapter 4: Stress Management Techniques

In today's fast-paced world, mastering stress management is vital for preserving overall well-being. This chapter digs into effective tactics to traverse the complicated environment of stress, offering you useful insights and concrete solutions.

Identifying and Addressing Stressors

Understanding the fundamental causes of stress is the first step toward managing it successfully. We cover many stressors, from work-related demands to personal issues, helping you identify and classify the causes of stress in your life. By recognizing these stresses, you obtain a greater perspective on how to handle and lessen their effect.

Mindful Stress Reduction Practices

Mindfulness acts as a potent antidote to the turmoil of everyday living. This section exposes you to mindfulness practices particularly tailored for stress reduction. From mindful breathing exercises to guided meditation, you'll discover practical strategies to create a present-moment awareness that may dramatically decrease stress. These techniques not only provide serenity to your mind but also strengthen your capacity to handle adversity with perseverance.

Creating Your Personalized Stress-Resilience Plan

No two persons experience stress in the same manner, and consequently, a one-size-fits-all approach to stress management is unhelpful. This section leads you through the process of developing a customized stress-resilience strategy suited to your requirements. Drawing on the insights acquired from recognizing stressors and adding mindful practices, you'll design a complete plan to build resilience and flourish in the face of life's obstacles.

As you begin on your path, examine your strengths, coping techniques, and favored hobbies. Your individualized plan will not only serve as a blueprint for stress management but also allow you to proactively handle stressors as they emerge.

In conclusion, Chapter 5 provides you with a comprehensive knowledge of stress management by digging into the identification and focused addressing of stressors, presenting mindfulness as an effective stress reduction technique, and helping you through the building of a tailored stress-resilience plan. By following these tactics, you are ready to take control of stress and cultivate a more balanced and meaningful existence.

Chapter 5: MindFit at Work: Integrating Wellness into Your Professional Life

In the fast-paced sphere of professional life, mastering the skill of overcoming workplace stress is crucial for sustained success and personal well-being. This chapter goes into practical techniques to handle pressures and build a healthy work environment.

Navigating Workplace Stress

The contemporary office is typically a crucible of pressure, deadlines, and high expectations. In this part, we discuss practical techniques for detecting and managing stress. From time management skills to creating a positive mentality, the objective is to provide workers with the tools required to flourish in high-demand situations. By identifying the origins of stress and employing appropriate coping methods, people may unleash their full potential without sacrificing mental health.

Incorporating MindFit Practices into Your Workday

MindFit techniques provide a comprehensive approach to promoting mental well-being. This section provides a range of mindfulness exercises, stress-reducing tactics, and productivity hacks meant to smoothly blend into the workplace. From short mindfulness sessions to strategic pauses, the objective is to encourage professionals to inject moments of peace into their everyday routines. By establishing a MindFit mentality, people may maximize their cognitive capacities, boost attention, and raise overall work performance.

Building a Mental Wellness Culture in Your Workplace: True change needs a communal effort. This section covers how executives and workers alike may contribute to building a mental health culture inside their firms. From leadership strategies that promote employee well-being to promoting open communication regarding mental health, the focus is on establishing an atmosphere where people feel supported and appreciated. By accepting a collaborative responsibility for mental well-being, companies may become not just more productive but also more empathetic and resilient.

In conclusion, Chapter 5 highlights the relevance of MindFit at Work, underlining the symbiotic link between personal well-being and professional success. By negotiating workplace stress, implementing MindFit practices, and developing a mental health culture, people and organizations may carve a road toward sustainable performance. This chapter offers a guide for professionals seeking not only success in their jobs but also satisfaction in their lives.

Chapter 6: MindFit for Students: Nurturing Mental Resilience in Academic Life

In the quest for academic success, students frequently encounter the tremendous obstacle of controlling stress. This chapter goes into comprehensive tactics aimed at reinforcing mental resilience, and helping students to handle the hard terrain of academic life with grace.

Strategies for Managing Academic Stress

Academic stress is an inherent aspect of student life, but efficient stress management is the key to sustaining mental well-being. Explore evidence-based practices such as time management, goal planning, and mindfulness to create a resilient mentality. By implementing these tactics into your academic practice, you may harness stress as a motivator rather than a deterrent, building a better connection with academic problems.

Balancing Academic and Personal Life

Achieving a good balance between academic endeavors and personal life is vital for continued well-being. This section addresses practical methods for time allocation, self-care, and boundary establishing. By finding the correct balance, students may enhance their academic achievement while nourishing their mental and emotional wellness. Learn to prioritize activities, build healthy habits, and make room for personal growth despite the pressures of academic commitments.

Creating a Supportive Student Community

No student should manage the intricacies of academic life in solitude. This chapter highlights the necessity of building a supportive student community. Explore options for cooperation, peer support, and mentoring to promote a feeling of belonging. Building a healthy network not only boosts academic experiences but also acts as a key foundation of emotional support. Learn how to create relationships, exchange experiences, and contribute to the establishment of a healthy and uplifting academic atmosphere.

In the overall path of academic and personal growth, this chapter acts as a compass, directing students toward the building of mental resilience.

By incorporating these methods into their everyday life, students may not only resist the stresses of academic obstacles but also emerge stronger, armed with the means to succeed in the evolving terrain of higher education.

Chapter 7: The MindFit Lifestyle: Sustaining Mental Wellness Long-Term

In the search for lasting mental well-being, Chapter 8 digs into the essence of building a MindFit lifestyle. The chapter provides detailed guidance on creating habits that not only boost immediate mental fitness but also set the basis for long-term psychological well-being. By grasping the subtleties of habit development, people may build sustainable routines that survive the test of time.

Establishing Habits for Ongoing Mental Fitness

This section discusses the science underlying habit development and its substantial influence on mental health. It highlights the relevance of persistent, constructive behaviors in creating resilience and reinforcing the mind against life's adversities. Readers are directed through practical methods to implement MindFit concepts into their everyday routines, converting them into habits that contribute to sustained mental health. By adopting deliberate behaviors, people may proactively manage stress, boost attention, and create a resilient attitude.

Adapting MindFit Principles to Different Life Stages

Life is a dynamic journey, distinguished by many phases and transformations. Chapter 8 highlights the necessity for adaptation in sustaining mental well-being throughout varied life periods. Whether managing the demands of a hectic job, raising a family, or approaching the golden years of retirement, the MindFit lifestyle remains relevant and flexible. This section presents specific insights and tactics for applying MindFit concepts to various life phases, ensuring that people may effortlessly incorporate mental well-being into the ever-evolving fabric of their lives.

Connecting with the MindFit Community for Continuous Support

Recognizing the significance of community in preserving mental well-being, this section underscores the necessity of creating relationships with like-minded people. The MindFit community offers a source of inspiration, motivation, and shared experiences. Readers are educated on how to connect with this supporting network, both online and offline, promoting a feeling of belonging and responsibility. By sharing accomplishments and problems within the MindFit community, people may magnify their commitment to mental well-being and draw strength from the collective knowledge of a supportive network.

In conclusion, Chapter 7 jhighlights the MindFit lifestyle as a dynamic and comprehensive approach to preserving mental fitness. Through the formation of deliberate habits, flexibility to life's many phases, and active participation with a supportive group, people may create a resilient mentality that survives the test of time. This chapter serves as a light of direction, motivating readers to embrace a lifetime path toward mental health, one conscious step at a time.

CONCLUSION

As we draw the curtains on your MindFit Mastery adventure, it's time to reflect on the steps you've achieved towards creating a robust and healthy mind. Throughout this transforming journey, you've used the power of self-awareness, mindfulness, and purposeful mental workouts to raise your cognitive ability.

In celebrating your MindFit Mastery journey, contemplate the enormous influence on your everyday life. The improved capacity to negotiate stress with grace, the heightened concentration that accelerates productivity, and the robust attitude that stands unshaken in the face of obstacles - these are the results of your devotion to mental fitness.

Remember, the trip doesn't finish here; it only develops. Continue to incorporate the MindFit concepts into your routine, strengthening the behaviors that have contributed to your mental well-being. Whether it's a regular mindfulness practice or participating in brain-boosting activities, make these aspects a permanent fixture in your life.

Moreover, share your MindFit discoveries with others. As you've observed directly, the ripple effect of a robust mind stretches beyond personal borders. By encouraging people around you, you contribute to a collective awareness of mental well-being, building a community that feeds on shared progress.

Embracing a Future of Abundant Mental Wellness:

As you go into the future, visualize a landscape loaded with the fruits of robust mental well-being.

Your MindFit Mastery journey has armed you with a toolset for managing the challenges of contemporary life with a deep feeling of balance and clarity.

In this future, stress is not a stumbling hurdle but a driver for progress. Challenges become chances for learning and growth, and failures are regarded as stepping stones towards a more robust and flexible mind. Your mental well-being is a cornerstone, providing a stable basis for the pursuit of your objectives and dreams.

Embrace a proactive attitude to mental well-being. Just as you would engage in physical fitness, dedicate time and attention to cultivating your mental wellness. Whether it's indulging in activities that offer you pleasure, practicing gratitude, or seeking expert help when required, these acts lead to a healthy and thriving mind.

Cultivate an attitude of constant improvement. The road toward rich mental well-being is dynamic, needing a commitment to continuing improvement. Be open to discovering new mindfulness approaches, remaining educated about the newest research on mental health, and modifying your tactics as required.

In this future, the advantages of your MindFit Mastery path extend well beyond personal fulfillment. As you exude a positive and resilient attitude, you become a light of inspiration for people around you. Your dedication to mental well-being not only affects your life but also has a ripple effect, impacting the well-being of your community and beyond.

In conclusion, enjoy the milestones of your MindFit Mastery journey and look forward to a future when mental well-being is not just a goal but a way of life. Through your continuing devotion and the sharing of your experiences, contribute to a society where abundant mental well-being is enjoyed by everyone.

Appendix

Additional Resources, Tools, and Worksheets

In this extensive appendix, we give a variety of supplemental resources aimed at improving your knowledge and application of the provided subject.

Resources:

Explore a handpicked collection of extra resources that go further into the major themes addressed. From scientific publications to informative blog entries, these resources serve as essential companions to improve your knowledge.

Tools:

Empower your trip with a series of carefully picked tools that boost your skill in executing the stated tactics. Whether you're seeking efficiency in data analysis or accuracy in project management, these tools are geared to boost your skills.

Worksheets:

The practical application sits at the core of learning. Utilize our painstakingly created worksheets to transform theoretical ideas into real outcomes. Each worksheet is purposefully intended to enhance your comprehension, creating a hands-on approach that strengthens your grasp of fundamental topics.

Frequently Asked Questions (FAQs)

Embark on a guided journey of the most prevalent questions regarding our material. Here, we resolve doubts, give explanations, and provide subtle insights to enable a comprehensive knowledge of the subject matter.

Q1: How do I optimize the usefulness of the new resources?

A1: The materials given are aimed at enhancing your learning experience. Start by examining items linked with your interests or areas of difficulty. Utilize them as extra reading to get other views and expand your comprehension.

Q2: Are the tools suggested compatible with multiple operating systems?

A2: Yes, the tools listed in our toolbox are picked for their flexibility. They cater to a range of operating systems, enabling accessibility across varied platforms. However, it's suggested to verify the current compatibility updates from the relevant tool suppliers.

Q3: How can I properly include the worksheets in my learning process?

A3: Approach the worksheets as practical activities to reinforce theoretical topics. Engage with them methodically, ensuring you implement the concepts stated. Use the worksheets as a dynamic tool to test your knowledge and enhance your abilities via hands-on practice.

Q4: Are there any special conditions for employing the increased resources?

A4: The materials appeal to a wide audience, and although some may presuppose baseline knowledge, they are typically accessible to learners at different levels. Be careful to study the necessary qualifications indicated beside each resource to determine its compatibility with your current skill level.

Q5: Can I offer more questions or request extra clarity on certain topics?

A5: Absolutely! We welcome your concerns and are devoted to establishing a friendly learning environment. Feel free to submit more questions, and our staff will swiftly respond to them, thus expanding your learning experience.

Navigate through our FAQ area for a comprehensive grasp of probable inquiries and receive clarification on complexities, allowing a smooth integration of our information into your learning experience.